No More Tears Left

Sian Treadwell

ISBN: 9798861105378

I DEDICATE THIS BOOK IN LOVING MEMORY
OF MY TWO ANGELS

TWO SURVIVORS, MY PARENTS & MY HUSBAND

CONTENTS

Acknowledgments

1   The beginning   Pg 7

2   What's next   Pg 11

3   Roller coaster   Pg 17

4   Would you believe it   Pg 25

5   Not again!   Pg 31

6   Funeral   Pg 37

7   What's incompetent cervix?   Pg 41

8   Well I never   Pg 45

9   To be continued …   Pg 54

10   About the author   Pg 53

ACKNOWLEDGMENTS

I'd like to thank my angels, my girls, husband &
parents for being my support and back bone.
Huge thank you to the staff at Addenbrookes
hospital especially Dr Hoveyda.

A thank you to Dr Christmas at Addenbrookes for
his support with my anxiety.
William Harvey hospital.

Penny Abatzi- Serum clinic Greece

Thank you to incompetent cervix UK support
group on Facebook.

Thank you to my brothers, sister in laws, nieces,
nephews, Julie, Caroline NICU nurses and lastly
thank you for reading.

xxxx

The beginning

"Where do you see yourself when you leave school?" that's the all-time question right?

Well my answer definitely wasn't to be a mum!

In fact at 14 years of age I was told, I would never be able to conceive naturally due to my periods not being regular, I could go 6 months to a year at times.

To say I wasn't bothered would be false, I was bothered but....too young to understand what that would entail, after all no one prepares you for it or for what your about to read.

18 years old I had qualified as a hair stylist aiming to own a salon was where I my all-time goal was. Already being in a long term relationship, renting a property, starting to live life after experiencing a tough time at school from bullies.

The world was my oyster.

I started to become very tired, upset tummy, thought to myself "oh no I've caught a bug…."

Strangely it started to last longer than a week, my mood was very up and down, weight gain was real,

My parents was getting ready for a big family and friends bbq when SHOCK hit!

Mum needed to pop out to get some extra bits, whilst out mum grabbed a pregnancy test. "what is that for?" I asked.

"You darling" mum calmly said.

"err no don't need that, I definitely not pregnant, the doctor said I couldn't too remember?" I stated

"yes Sian but just rule it out" mum insisted.

Off we trot home, and boom there it was, a BIG solid positive, my knees went to jelly and first thought was "How am I going to tell my dad?"

I cried, shut myself in bathroom, felt like I couldn't breathe, just kept asking myself "how, in disbelief"

My mum on the other hand, as calm as a mouse said "I thought so, I just had a feeling"

Well mystic meg I didn't have a clue and was absolutely sh*tting myself!

All I can say is from that day onwards my mum never left my side, she's my rock, my go to, my turn to, without her I don't know where I would be.

Also she had to break the news to my dad… I was so worried about telling him, but he also has been the most supportive dad ever, I'll always be his little girl. Every day I count my blessings.

So after a couple of day pass my mum advised me to book the doctors, simply thinking I was just a few weeks, well here comes shock number two… I was 9 and 1/2 weeks, was not expecting that!

So after both shocks settled I started to tell family and friends, by this point excitement started to kick in.

My pregnancy was tough, I had severe sickness and constant low blood pressure making me feel extremely light headed. But baby was doing fantastic and that's all I was concerned about.

20 weeks arrived I was starting to feel flutters, they were so cute!

Itching to find out what I was having . . . ITS….A GIRL!

Well we non stopped shopped for her, her wardrobe was out doing us all.

Then at 23 weeks my world fell apart, it was couple of weeks before Christmas, out shopping with my parents when I kept having strange feelings, not pain as such but it did stop me in my walks.

I went home and thought maybe baby was pushing down hard on my pelvis, early house I became more uncomfortable, still believing baby was laying difficult.

7am I couldn't take it anymore, so I called the maternity ward, a midwife asked a few questions then said "take some paracetamol, I don't believe it anything to worry about, your very early, if you still worried called back in couple of hours"

Within 10 minutes the midwife called back and said "Sian I think you should come in, just to check all is ok which I'm sure it is"

So off we go. Still extremely uncomfortable (no pain)

Arrived safely to a midwife who led me into a room applying the monitor on me to check on baby girl, with minutes she came rushing in to ask to examine me.

At this point I'm panicking "what is happening!"

Mum was holding me hand.

Midwife examined

. "Your 7cms dilated, we need to take you to theatre NOW" Nurse demanded whilst alarming further medical staff.

"but wait I'm only 23 weeks" FEAR was striking me "what does that mean?" body uncontrollably shaking.

So many faces coming into the theatre room, the neonatal care team getting for my baby, consultants trying to explain my babies chance of surviving, which wasn't much….

TEARS were filling, FEAR rushing through, ANXIETY through the roof, people everywhere, my mother being my birthing partner, staying strong for her daughter, but I could see the worry in her eyes…words just can't explain.

Dad awaiting outside, brothers driving from all ends of the UK rushing to get to the hospital, awaiting news.

The birth itself was a roller coaster, where baby girl was so small from being so early she was feet first, and she got stuck, my placenta came away causing her lack of oxygen and she was born not breathing.

"wow writing this is harder than I thought"

"still feels like yesterday, the trauma is raw even though its 16 years this year" (2023)

After the neonatal team resuscitated her, they whisked her off very sharply. More baby consultants came in to talk to me to tell me she was extremely poorly.

I'll be honest I was in a whirl wind shock and was adamant she was going to be ok.

I wasn't allowed to see her, every hour went passed all I wanted was to see her, especially when I was put on a ward with all women who had given birth but all had their babies with them, visiting time arrived and their families all cooing over their precious babies, whilst I lay there not knowing if mine was going to survive.

My parents got me moved as I just couldn't stop the tears streaming, once moved the hospital vicar offered to christen baby girl, to which I named her Morgan and was given a bit more hope that my baby will put a good fight up. My gorgeous dainty 1lb8ozs girl. Longing to hold her.

Hours past into early hours finally I was able to see Morgan, excited and scared I was wheeled down.

No words can prepare you for the neonatal journey, machines bleeping everywhere, staff whizzing around, very poorly babies, a roller coaster was in store.

I spent a few hours with Morgan when a neonatal nurse told me to go and rest, she would call if needed to.

I wasn't going back on the ward with the new mothers and babies so I discharged myself, living only 10 minutes down the road, it felt right.

Off I went reluctant to leave baby girl.

Couple of hours sleep, up I jumped, fully dressed, washed, hair brushed I just couldn't wait to see Morgan, I didn't have a call so there me thinking "no news is good news"

SHOCK, that wasn't the case, arrived in the hospital to be called into a room with lots of medical staff to be told,

"Morgan has had bleeds on the brain, we need you to make a decision, to switch her life support off and let her drift away. Or keep her going on support but now she won't have a normal life, she is brain dead."

F*ck me did the tears stream, I actually couldn't even talk, I was given time to make a decision.

"Hardest decision ever to be made!!"

18 years old and been given that decision. My faults "why me, why her" praying to god for a miracle cure, but knowing it was too late.

Well put it this was my view was… what quality of life will she have, I'll be selfish to make her live a life she won't enjoy. That was my opinion, so with the most shattered heart we turned her life support off with my parents, brothers and sister in laws around her incubator.

Morgan didn't pass straight away, she gave it a good go, the most loveliest neonatal nurses Caroline and Julie were incredible, you could see they were hurt by it too, they really made such a sad heart breaking time, memorable.

Caroline and Julie gave Morgan a little bath, dressed er in baby born outfit, spoke to her, wrapped her up in the cutest blanket, done her hand and footprints.

Then all the family got a cuddle with Morgan who's heart was still beating all the way round till she got to me, then she passed away.

Guess the saying is right "they know their mummy"

Myself and parents walked Morgan to the chapel where a little Moses basket waited for her, I just couldn't bear to look, eyes swollen, tears streaming, voice speechless.

Mum gently laid her down with a kiss.

All heart broken, she laid peacefully.

Nothing can prepare you for a death of a child.

Christmas was meant to be a time of joy, cheer and laughter.

There was me crying, grieving, lost, hating Christmas, wishing for my baby girl back, hating my body, wondering what I did wrong!

Why me?

WHATS NEXT?

"You need to organize a funeral!"

Planning a funeral for a baby you held for 30 minutes, not even knowing how to plan a funeral. Just sitting crying, not having a clue of what I was doing, shut myself off to the world, never letting go of Morgan's piglet blanket that came out of the incubator, how was I to even able to talk to anyone to book my baby girls funeral….. I was meant to be planning a christening!

Truth be told I tried small little outings (outings I mean a supermarket shop) and I just couldn't do it, people would either say "you ok?"
My instant response "no" with tears streaming uncontrollably.
Comments you could hear from people judging "A young woman is walking around with a teddy" (little did they know it was piglet which had Morgan's smell on it and was only thing I had left of her)
The most upsetting for me was seeing families with their little miracles, wishing that was me pushing the pram, as much as I was happy for them,,
My heart shattered into pieces.
Going out was a daily reminder of grief!
The funeral I just couldn't face at the time. However truth be told I wish I was given a few more days and planned it because looking back it wasn't a goodbye I had planned, my plans was her future but never goodbye was I prepared for!

The funeral took place just days before Christmas. Yes this is the reason I struggle at Christmas, every angel you saw whether be poster, advert, billboard, picture. I saw that as my little angel my daily reminder of what I had lost. A part of me gone forever.

After the funeral the grief really set in, by this point I felt everyone had just moved on and forgotten Morgan. I felt like it was just me carrying the pain.

My parents I know felt my pain and allowed me to grieve my own way as one of their babies had sadly lost their life many years before my appearance, very different to Morgan, their baby was born with spina bifida.

They understood my pain, although its heart breaking losses it grew us closer. I am forever grateful for my parents, when I say I'd be lost without them, I sincerely mean it, through every storm they have been my rainbow.

A few months past…. Did it get easier?
Hell no!
 Do you learn to live with the pain?
Yes! Eventually.
Do you have daily reminders?
Yes!

It does make you stronger though, keeping strong is a big fight in life when your world has shattered, every breath you start to feel lucky for, every dream you had you try to make come true.

"!Do you have any thought in becoming a mum again?"
Nope!
Why? Because she was my life!
My relationship was rocky, we grieved in very different ways.

A very rare outing, as drinking booze just brang raw emotions back. I started to feel light headed, little bit of nausea.

Little did I know I was pregnant again, this time though, I was shocked whilst instantly feeling like I had been gifted.

This time I had found out I was pregnant about 8 weeks, every day I felt grateful for.

Pregnancy itself was tough, sickness was rife.

I did manage to find a few tips and tricks that helped.

Ready salted crisp's, very salted chip's from the chippy, cheese and tomato pizza.

Was it healthy?
No!
 Did it work?
YES!

Anything to keep sickness at bay, to enable me to eat my 5 a day in between.

Baby was happy and healthy that was my main focus.

So this time round I was given a red note maternity book (meaning high risk pregnancy in the UK)

I anxiously awaited my consultant appointment (which actually was my consultant who delivered Morgan)

So there's me trying to stay positive, of course my mum was there.

Running through my previous experience, tears filling, anxiety rushing through, panic attacks coming in fast.

Questions ready to ask.

Consultant lifts his head from my maternity notes and states " No need to worry it won't happen again, things happen like this and there's not always a reason."

I'm stunned like… huh? There's got to be a reason, things don't just happen!

Mum's looking confused, asking questions. By this point I'm zoned out not hearing as I'm so confused.

We left the appointment phoned family and remained positive.

As time went the excitement hit again, I finally built the confidence to unpack all Morgan's gorgeous outfits, cot etc.

Painted her room, my artistic dad done a piglet moral on the wall, it was incredible!

BOOM! Week 23 hit I was in town just casually walking around on a mother and daughter shopping day. I turned to mum. "mum I got a weird feeling low down"

"How does it feel? Is it painful?" mum asked

"No mum, not painful, it's weird."

Instantly mum demanded we call the hospital just to get checked out.

A week after finding out I was having another gorgeous girl.

Well….. I'm forever grateful she did make me call!

 I was in LABOUR again!!!!

Do to my previous the hospital agreed to see me straight away, as I arrived it was very calm, my midwife said "I'm just going to examine make sure all is well"

Well I'm lying there thinking, No it won't be happening again my

consultant said it wouldn't!
How wrong was he!!!…. and I…
I was dilating! I cried and cried here we go again, I'll burying another baby.
Mum holding my hand, calling my dad.
Medical staff rushing around.
I felt sick to the stomach, this time not just from morning sickness.

After what felt a lifetime (it was a few minutes) a midwife came to my side wiping my tears and said "We need to transfer you to a higher graded hospital for baby, as baby needs higher care if born now"
"where are you sending me, am I going to bury another baby?"
"hopefully not no, we will get you to a hospital prepared, possibly Manchester"
"Manchester? Oh no, please don't let me go alone" at this point I'm shaking so hard the beds shaking, I wasn't allowed to stand up, I had to have my head lower than my feet, feeling dizzy from being on the tilt, staff in and out checking me.

"Right Sian we have found you a bed, you are going to be blue lighted all the way, mum can go with you and a midwife, in-case you deliver on route, she's just getting her essentials together."

"i have nothing on me, where are we going, Manchester? "my voice croaking.
"No we managed to find a bed closer, you're going to a hospital in Kent"

By this point my dad was already at the hospital with a bag ready to follow the ambulance.
I was taken sharply into the ambulance tilted with blue lights all the way, Dartford bridge was closed whilst we was escorted over by police.
Yes apologies to the drivers held up that day.
 Dad got held up in the traffic but he arrived shortly after us. Bless him he was so worried, mum updated him when she could, thank god for mobile phones.

 Arrived swiftly this part is a bit of a blur, I was closely monitored, the staff was incredible, after a few discussions a team of consultants came together and decided to do an emergency McDonald suture (cervical stitch) as they managed to slow my labour down, to point it was classed as steady.
My anxiety by now was uncontrollable the medical team was so supportive specially being young, they bent a couple of rules to keep me calm. My anaesthetist even took his time to give me a spinal block that only numbed my bum and not all my legs, (a fear of mine is numb legs due to my panic

attacks)
Not only that they allowed my mum in the theatre, it made such a difference I felt SAFE. We spoke about getting a McDonald's after, I was starving! No pain felt just a little tugging and pulling, all normal.
 After recovery I was taken on to a ward, it was so clean and fresh, they booked a local hotel for my dad to stay, mum was allowed with me.
Couple of days being monitored I was itching to go out and walk. The team allowed me to the hotel where I managed a little snooze and freshen up.
Further days went by I was still stable, I insisted the staff for me to go home. The staff agreed and wrote a plan of action in my notes. I was strictly informed "due to your stitch it will be harder to tell labour, but you need to prevent it tearing, it will be harder to tell, but every day counts"

The plan was to go on home bed rest, if tightening's become frequent (pattern) any bleeding, pains etc go to hospital and be transferred back. Notes stated that.

A few days went by I had a home midwife (I had met her a few times at the local clinic when I was pregnant with Morgan) Keeping a diary of any tightening's, I managed to get to 26 weeks 4 days, my local midwife came to visit and felt a tighten and advised me to get checked.

Off I trot, notes was handed in, everything was spoken about again and again, I was refused transfer and placed on monitor for contractions, my tightening's was low down, I had very small bump yet staff insisted to keep putting them higher up. Due to this error they failed to pick up my contractions, by this point you could physically see my tummy tighten, I was starting to feel very uncomfortable, staff refused anyone to be with me, midwives wouldn't even help me to the toilet, I couldn't stand let alone walk.
Struggling to the toilet. Now on 26 weeks 6 days early hours I cried for help. A nurse reluctantly took me and there I just bled bright red. I shouted out knowing what the previous hospital had told me. The nurse said "its fine get in bed and go to sleep!"
"No please listen this isn't good, get my mum please, PLEASE!" begging with tears hardly standing, fearing my life and baby's life.
I was taken back to my bed on the ward and told to sleep.
Hours past feeling like days, I was literally hanging of the bed in so much pain. The woman next to me kept telling me to "shut up, stop moaning" kept complaining to the nurses about me.
8am day after bonfire night my mum was allowed in.

She came in to the site of me hanging off the bed, crying, trying to say I can't do this.

Mum ran out and demanded a doctor. 10 minutes later a doctor came in looked at my stomach and said "its Braxton hicks"

My mums eyes rolled "Sian's hanging off the bed in pain, you can see her stomach going rock hard, she has a stitch in, READ HER NOTES!"

Doctor said the monitors aren't picking up, we will try monitor again. Fact is monitor was placed to high up, more for a term time labour. I had a very small bump.

20 minutes later

"MUM I NEED TOO PUSH!!"

"Sian, NO, don't push I'll get help! Mum ran and screamed "SHE NEEDS TO PUSH!"

A nurse came in with a wheelchair as she did… A huge GUSH!

My waters broke… I was lifted off the bed quickly and wheeled to a delivery theatre where I had to wait to have my stitch cut.

 Trying so hard not to push but naturally my body was. A midwife rushed the doctor to cut the stitch and literally seconds later baby number two arrived with a little cry, sounded like a little meow.

 Neonatal team at the ready. I hadn't even noticed they was in the room, all prepared whisked baby off to neonatal.

 Whilst baby was cared for I had midwives congratulating me.

My only thoughts were ….. Why are they congratulating me?

She's too early, I'm going to lose her.

I just couldn't help but feel negative, what's meant to be an exciting and happy time, I felt alone, lost, started to hate my body and just thinking here we go again.

Shall I contact the funeral directors?

Roller coaster

As evening dawned I was approached by the hospital vicar (who had christened Morgan in the hospital) She couldn't believe it happened again, in just 11 months from Morgan's delivery/passing.

After hours past, which felt like days. My baby was stable enough for me to see her.
 First look at her and I just feel in love, small tiny 2lb8oz, fragile baby, fighting to stay alive.
 Being back in NICU frightened me, brung back all the horrific memories and heartache from before, gave me shivers, the noises from the machines sending me into panic attacks.
 I just couldn't take my eyes off her as I was wondering if this minute/hour would be the last time I got with her.
Every minute I counted as a blessing that she was still with us fighting every way she possibly could!
The strength within premature babies is beyond words, true natural fighters.

There was nothing to prepare me for the journey ahead.

I stayed with Mackenzie till early hours and discharged myself from the ward as I just wanted to be by her side.
The staff looking after Mackenzie was two incredible nurses who had looked after Morgan, Caroline and Julie
I Knew Mackenzie was in great hands so I headed home to get a couple of hours sleep, as Mackenzie was showing positive signs.

A couple of days past Mackenzie was doing fantastic!
Then we had a setback, unfortunately she had caught a nasty infection

(common with tiny fragile babies but also life threatening)
Very touch and go few days, Mackenzie being put on life support was an image I will never ever forget, I just prayed and prayed for a miracle. Staring at her lifeless body. I begged "Please don't leave me, I can't do life without you!"
I cried so long my eyes swollen.

Every minute counts in NICU, every hand wash, every precaution to prevent all the little fighters from getting poorly.
I never knew anything before Morgan and Mackenzie about premature babies, I was shocked. Was a huge eye opener.

In NICU they have a little kitchen where parents of premature's, poorly babies can have lunch or cup of tea, or even just a 5 minute break. On route there's a corridor filled with miracle's who had survived and went on to achieving huge milestones.
This was my hope on the dark days. I longed to get to that stage.
It was such a lovely touch.

Mackenzie fought so hard she started coming out the other side, came off life support back on cpap.
Cpap is a breathing equipment that just helps supports babies breathing, on cpap they are on the way to breathing for themselves it has different levels to which they get weaned off gradually, to which some go onto oxygen or fully breath themselves.
Incredible!

Once Mackenzie was fully over her infection, I managed to have my first cuddle, skin to skin, was the best cuddle in the world, I felt so lucky!
Tubes were everywhere from the monitors and cpap she was connected to but I wasn't worried on the nurse placed her on me, I had longed to hold her.
 I didn't want to put her down but to prevent germs and her getting cold, I had to hand her back to the nurse.
 As she become stronger day by day I started to get excited thinking yes she will be able to come home soon.
 Nurses said grandparents were welcome to come meet Mackenzie, I was so excited. We was allowed two at a time so the plan was I went in with mum whilst dad had a cuppa. Then mum swapped with dad.
 Eager to meet their granddaughter properly they arrived swiftly.

 Then disaster struck!
This time I was being told "Mackenzie is extremely poorly we are not sure

if she will make it, she needs to go on life support and have blood transfusion.

My world, my plans, started to fall to pieces.

"Why o why?"

"was it because I held her?" I couldn't help but think it was me that caused it, even though I took every precaution.

Whilst medical staff tried to stabilize Mackenzie. Myself and parents awaited in the tea room in silence, every person who walked past we would pause in breath wondering if nurse was coming to tell us there was nothing they could do.

No words can describe that anxious helpless wait.

A lovely lady who came to visit her little fighter spoke to me. Wiping my tears she was telling me

"this is the NICU roller coaster. One minute they are on top form the next they are whizzing downhill very quickly, as quick as they fall they also bounce back just as quick, stay strong"

The lady was great informing me of groups and websites where other parents who was on the NICU roller coaster can talk with each other who fully understood the emotions.

I was a bit worried speaking about my journey as my loss of Morgan I never liked to talk about. If anyone asked if I had more children I always said yes two.

I couldn't bring myself to say one in NICU one in heaven, just thinking it made me cry. Even to this day

Finally a nurse came in and said we was able to see her, explaining what had been done and that a doctor will be coming to take more bloods to see if the antibiotics were working.

My mum and I went in to the NICU room, ensuring we had showered in hand gel.

After a short 5 minutes the doctor came to take the bloods, I felt like I needed to pull myself together, I don't like needles specially on my little girl.

Off I went back to the tea room and I said dad you go with mum I just need take some time out to pull myself together.

All of I sudden I hear my mum shouting, running up the corridor.

A bit dazed trying to gasp what was going on. Mackenzie's monitors going off, nurses rushing to her aid. Mum distraught.

Medical staff started doing resuscitation closing the curtains around Mackenzie's incubator.

I howled, mum was in pieces, dad was trying to comfort her tearing up himself.

We was guided back into the tea room being told a doctor will come in shortly.

Well that really did feel like forever. My mum stepped outside the tea room door to speak with a passing nurse her voice shaking with emotion.

My mum had witnessed suffocation to Mackenzie from the doctor taking her bloods. No wonder she screamed out.

The doctor was rushing around, knowing Mackenzie was on life support and where the tube was laid she still went to tube side, reached out and pulled Mackenzie's leg over not realizing she was kinking the life support tube.

Mum was watching and explained she saw Mackenzie's little body struggle, mum shouted at the doctor "THE BABY!!"

The Doctor just looked and carried on still oblivious, a nurse across the room seeing to another little fighter, noticed the monitor readings dropping dramatically, she ran over and shouted at the doctor, taking instant control.

Mum explained all sudden staff was everywhere, and that's when I came running and saw resuscitation being performed.

Instantly I thought that's it, she's dead!

The doctor came to apologize but being brutally honest I didn't want to hear it, I couldn't hear it, my concern was my baby.

How can "mistakes" be made that potentially can cause end of life.

I know mistakes can happen and staff are overworked and most are exhausted but making these mistakes are deadly and can rip someone's world apart in seconds. For the time you can take to keep yourself focused would be more practically than over doing it making wrong moves, which could harm more than just yourself.

"What does this mean now?"

Still waiting for an update, pacing the room. Mum unable to relax, dad with his head in his hand looking down.

Eventually we was told they had managed to stabilize Mackenzie again, this time a different doctor had taken bloods correctly and we was awaiting to see the infection levels hopefully start dropping.

From this day onwards I never left her side, occasionally I would pop outside the door for max of 5 mins for fresh air. I hardly slept but when I did I could hear the monitors in my sleep bleeping.

Hours felt like days, days felt like weeks, weeks felt like months.

With many ups and downs.

8 weeks past and Mackenzie was moved to a cot. This was HUGE! I was able to dress her, change her mum, pick her up for cuddles, I could actually start feeling like a mummy.

Bonding with your baby in NICU is the hardest emotional struggle. I personally struggled, I adored her so much but felt so helpless many times I felt I failed her.
A couple of days in a cot and completely off cpap but on low oxygen the nurse said "shall we try feeding her?"
"Definitely!" I said smiling heart pounding with excitement.
The nurse gave the first bottle to ensure Mackenzie was taking it correctly.

I felt like my firsts of parenting was stolen, but I knew it was all for correct reasons, the nurses had ways of knowing if baby was correctly sucking the bottle, swallowing so that was enough to know it was right.
First bottle Mackenzie whizzed it down, the bottle was tiny but looked huge against her little face.
The Nurse was great with her, and said "your one step closer to home now, once feeding is sussed, there's no stopping you"
My heart skipped a beat, I couldn't wait to call mum and tell her home is Insite.
From then all I had multiple little meets with medicals staff arranging all the correct home care. Due to Mackenzie being unable to come off oxygen completely we had oxygen delivered and set up at home.
Lots of restrictions came with home oxygen, not allowed near radiators due to the heat. Not to touch cooking oils then the baby as tubes can react. The tubes weren't overly long so weren't able to just walk about into different rooms.
Still when these were installed and I was given a transit one the excitement whizzed through I just couldn't contain it.

Mum scrubbed the house top to bottom, dad finished the baby room and set the pram up. It was all falling into place.

A week before home time, I arrived a hospital.
Went into the NICU room where Mackenzie had been for 11 weeks and she wasn't there.
I questioned the staff and was told to wait in the tea room.

Here we go, they are going to tell me she's not coming home. This NICU journey is one hell of a rollercoaster.

A nurse came in and explained a baby had come in with a disease that can make other babies extremely poorly sometimes death.

Its passed on by touch.

Somehow (I'm still puzzled to this day) Mackenzie had contracted it which then meant she had to be isolated in a room on her way and gowns for anyone entering the room had to be worn, along with gloves and mask.

"So I can't touch my own baby?"

"You can but you can't come out the room wearing the gown you need to dispose and thoroughly wash hands before leaving." nurse explained

This is odd. And felt extremely lonely. I wasn't able to chat to other parents only wave through a window. Mackenzie on her own in a large room, it saddened me.

Luckily though the disease didn't affect her, her soiled nappies just had to be disposed in a certain bin as this was also a way from the disease passing contact.

"PHEW" that was such a relief that she remained healthy.

Week 12 arrived and guess what!!!

YES! I got to bring the car seat in and take my baby home!

The long wait was over, I get to cuddle lots, I get to be a full time mummy, to watch you grow and protect you forever!

Having her on home oxygen was very scary but we soon got the hang of it.

We still had a long road ahead with many hospital appointments, frequent baby weigh in clinics.

Baby milk was on a prescription so a weekly trip to the chemist too.

These felt like a breeze to what we had already gone through.

Every person that met Mackenzie said she was like a little doll.

Her cries was soft, in fact she hardly cried, so content and happy. Most luckiest woman.

As the years went by her character of strength shone through, loved by everyone who met her, kind, funny and brave. She loved life.

Being Premature at such an early stage having weakness in her lungs (chronic lung disease) did mean that a normal cold to us really took toll on Mackenzie. Often turning into pneumonia, she suffered with croup where an air ambulance landed.

As much as we protected her when she started preschool was mainly the time the bugs started. luckily Mackenzie always fought hard and medical care was quick to help get her back fighting fit.

Having Chronic lung disease just didn't stop her, sometimes slowed her down when came to running (still does at times) she never let it phase her of stop her.

My gorgeous miracle who not only is the strongest girl I know but she is who made mummy stronger.

A lady once said to me "Do you know Morgan is in Mackenzie, that's why she loves life!"

These words have always stuck with me and from then on I always saw it. Those words helped me with my grieving, the strength was not only Mackenzie but her sister pushing her to keep going.

After Mackenzie and Morgan, people used to always say "you having anymore?"

My head wanted to say "yes! I'd like a football team!" My goal in life was to succeed, provide and live.

However my HEART was NO, I don't think I can handle it.

I kept telling myself it's ok I'd be well looked after because of the history and surely it couldn't happen again?

Remember this line "SURELY THIS CAN'T HAPPEN AGAIN!?"

To be honest with you although I was asked daily, it was also out of my mind, I was fully focused on how lucky I was to have Mackenzie and how every milestone hit was remarkable!

Every day my famous words were "that's my girl!" "I'm so proud of you"

When you have lost and then a near loss you cherish every moment, every second is a blessing.

Not many people will understand this if they haven't experienced loss, they look at you like you over dramatic.

At this point all I will say is….. Don't allow someone's judgement to affect how you feel as a parent.

Unless they hear words from you, they have no right to side and judge.

Not everyone has an easy start to parenting, not every parenting role is easy.

Every parent have different morals, its team work that makes the dreams work. (not speaking just relationships but support around)

Single parents still make it work but hearsay doesn't give single parents enough credit because they only hear one side. Again judgement is yet a fail.

Through loss and pregnancy you learn who your mates and family are.

Slowly you become unimportant in people's lives, you will only be important to the ones who care.

I was a young mum but I don't carry any regrets, how it happened, yes I wasn't married or financially stable but life sometimes doesn't work out the way you plan.

So you pick yourself up, wipe your tears, straighten your crown and you own it.

Grieving is one of the hardest emotions because you never get over it, you just learn to live with it, not a day goes by where you don't think. I WONDER WHAT LIFE WOULD BE LIKE?

Every celebration whether it be Christmas, birthdays you just wish they was there and imagine what it would be like.

Although I felt extremely lucky Mackenzie fought for her life and made it, I did carry guilt on Morgan, but Mackenzie helped me to live for tomorrow, never took anything for granted, made every day happy memories.

Every milestone Mackenzie reached was miracle that is where you looked back and saw how far we all came.

WOULD YOU BELIEVE IT

Watching Mackenzie grow was the best feeling in the world.
Her laughter contagious, she brightens every room she enters, her character shining through. Her love for life beyond words.

I was never thinking of more children, I felt unsure, I had thoughts that I never wanted to have an only child but it was never a certainty as life itself was very unpredictable.
With having 3 older brothers myself with a large age gap, growing up it felt a little lonely, so I always had in mind that maybe one day I will but it was never the plan at the time.
  I was on pill when fell poorly with urine infection and was given antibiotics.
I never knew that being on antibiotics prevents your pill working fully.
Can you guess what I'm about to say??

You got it another unexpected surprise! Another baby on the way!

This time was a little more complicated as I had Mackenzie, I still wasn't fully settled in life, and of course had BIG concerns of what was to come in this pregnancy.

 Having Mackenzie the weeks were flying due to all her social commitments, play dates, my work, actually looking back it was a good distraction.
Once I found out I booked the doctors for as soon as possible knowing I was high risk I just didn't want to delay any care or take chances that could result in another loss.

My GP at the time was very understanding with allowing me to choose a different hospital due to my previous bad experiences.

Before I continue I will say this is my own personal story of events some people had gone to have amazing experiences at the hospital which I unfortunately didn't. Every pregnancy and experience is different as you can probably tell even mine have been different.

The first hospital choice I wanted I was talked out of but at time the reasons the GP was saying made sense.

My first choice hospital was over an hour's drive at time so if I did go into preterm labour I wasn't sure I'd make it.

London hospitals was also a mention but again it's the travelling if preterm labour happens again, although of course that was not what we was wanting.

Doctor made me aware that I needed to choose a hospital within good distance as I would have regular appointments to.

So now a new local hospital was picked my GP wrote to a specialist consultant, with my pregnancy history.

Within a couple of weeks I had an appointment with the consultant to run through my notes and the plan.

Before attending my appointment I had spoken to a few medical staff from different areas and all said I recommend you ask for a cervical suture (a stitch)   The team at William Harvey in Kent had said I should have had a stitch early with Mackenzie no chances should have been taken.

Cervical suture was like what I had in an emergency with Mackenzie, this time would be done around 12 weeks.

My mum and I done a bit of research and wrote some questions down in preparation for the consultant.

Arriving to the appointment I was feeling slightly excited, trying to stay positive with built up anxiety trying to take away.

"Sian Treadwell the Dr will see you now"

Suddenly the anxiety won, my heart started to race awaiting the unknown.

"Hi please take a seat, so tell me what brings you here?" consultant asked.

"well I have gone into labour at 23 weeks twice. Ones passed one survived. With my survivor I had emergency stitch which stretched me a couple more weeks. I'm pregnant again and researched that a cervical suture is advised, no risks should be taken."

"Yes I see" consultant said reading through my notes "well I don't advise a stitch, I think you had a infection that caused preterm, so we will start you on antibiotics, along with a cream to insert into your vagina and in 6 weeks we will start you on cyclogest pessaries to insert once of an evening when you go to bed."

I was very taken back by the consultant response, I just wasn't prepared at this point, so my mum spoke to the consultant stating our concerns and explained that we feel a cervical suture would be the route and it's the way we want to go.

"No, I've made my decision. Please book your next appointment in 2 weeks at the front desk." consultant said abruptly.

Walking out I just had sheer panic, anxiety and fear.

Confused as to why I was refused, concerns of is it going to happen again?

He mentioned infection, yet I'd had swaps when ii had my previous pregnancies no one ever mentioned an infection caused labour.

Mum and I both baffled kept going over trying to understand but it just never made sense.

However we came to the decision to trust the consultant as after all he was fully trained/qualified. we aren't experts within pregnancies, labour etc.

Every two weeks I had to go to the consultants clinic. To be honest that did make me feel like I was being cared for, I mean what really can happen within two weeks?

12 weeks pregnant I felt on top of the world, no morning sickness occasionally felt nausea but rarely was. I started having weird cravings for steak and BBQ ribs, they was never really my go to foods but it was all I wanted.

I started to show really early in this pregnancy so I started to tell family the news as I struggled to hide the bump.

Week 14 swiftly came round, I went to my appointment which seem positive.

I felt good, I was on all the medicines, Mackenzie was healthy, all was looking good.

Two days passed I went to the loo in preparation of having an early chilled night, Mackenzie was tucked up in bed, my parents on their evening stroll, when suddenly I felt really strange like a gush.

I looked down and the toilet was bright red.

In total shock I couldn't get out the toilet quick enough! I grabbed my phone and called my parents crying.

"MUM, MUM please come home hurry!!! I'm bleeding, I'm losing my baby!!"

"We are coming, call an ambulance" mum trying to stay calm.

"what's the number?" in total shock my mind had gone blank.

"999 Sian, try stay calm" mum trying to reassure me but I could tell she was worried.

I sat on the stairs near the front door awaiting the ambulance. Shaking like a leaf.

Luckily I hadn't even thought to flush the toilet which helped the ambulance crew to get an estimate of how much blood I had lost.

Parents arrived just as the ambulance crew was explaining I needed to be taken int hospital as I was possibly having a miscarriage.

Cor did I cry!

Luckily I was able to have mum with me whilst my dad listened out for Mackenzie at home.

I was put on a ward to be monitored awaiting a scan.

Still bleeding I was simply preparing for the words we can't find a heartbeat. Worried about how I was going to tell Mackenzie.

Hating my body for yet again letting me down.

Then

A portable scan machine was wheeled to my bedside.

"Hi Sian I'm just going to have a look at baby, see what's going on, your still bleeding, is that correct?

"yes" I said bluntly, anxiously waiting, it honestly felt like it was taking hours. Truth was it was literally minutes.

"Sian can you see? The sonographer turning the screen to mum and I.

"Yes" I responded.

"Baby seems happy, there's a strong heartbeat" she said smiling "Everything looks as it should."

"So why am I bleeding, what's causing it?" I said relieved.

"Sometimes there's no explanation, it can just happen." she reassured me.

Shortly after I was released to go home. Naturally I thought I had better rest more, do moderate bed rest, which was hard having Mackenzie running around.

My following consultant appointment came round and I explained what happened whilst he was running through my notes.

The consultant explained sometimes there's no reason for bleeds, they are common.

From here the consultant requested another scan, and booked me to have an internal cervix scan, to measure cervix to ensure it hadn't thinned or dilated.

During the scan the sonographer was taking many measurements ensuring everything was as it should be and baby was happy.

All seemed good no signs of anything of a concern.

Couple weeks on I was feeling great. Even felt great within myself. The glowing stage in pregnancy I actually never believed people when they said you will be glowing soon lol, I never glowed with my girls!
This time was very different.
I was in a wheelchair to go round shops, resting as much as I could, when I could, as I was worried that too much walking would send me into labour, trying everything in my willpower to prevent anything to stress my body.

I woke up from a nap with Mackenzie and felt odd.
I went to the loo and there it was another bleed.
Called hospital who said I was to come in due to history. Arrived, checked and away back home I was sent.
My consultant was informed the next day and he said "you are likely to bleed throughout your pregnancy, it's probably your normal"
I responded "thing is this is my third pregnancy and never happened before? So I wouldn't say it's my normal."
I kept over thinking this conversation in my head…. surely bleeding is not normal in pregnancy?
Still do this day I'm baffled.

Bleeding lasted as few days, I was feeling baby movements which was reassuring, constantly counted the kicks.

Week 20 arrived wow I was really showing now! No hiding it what so ever. My pregnancy with my girls I didn't look pregnant but this time was like I swallowed a basketball.
Went along for my normal 20 weeks scan and wowzah.
"ITS A BOY!" sonographer said.

I did have a gut feeling I was expecting boy because I felt so different to my previous and actually felt glamorous, but same time it was a shock to actually hear it.
Well I was straight to buying blue, so excited by this time. Name was thought of in seconds of the news, I could not find another girls name at time.

Constantly thinking wow it's going to be so nice. Mackenzie was told (although she was very young to understand) but she shouted "BROTHER" which was cute and picked some lovely teddies for him.
I started planning the room with Mackenzie's help, I felt I needed to include her in everything. You always worry you child will feel left out, I actually don't know why we worry about it because none of us mums or dads would, but it's a natural feeling we all have.

The love for your kids are beyond words.

Preparing for the next chapter was so exciting.

I felt like I was really prepared and organized, just starting to prepare my hospital bag, not thinking I was going into labour any time soon, as consultant told me it wouldn't happen.

Just pure excitement.

NOT AGAIN!

The excitement soon turned to doom!!

Week 23 yet again, this time I actually felt great still, but yet I was ROBBED.

In the evening I went to the loo and saw the plug (the plug is a blood mixed discharge which is laying on the whole of cervix as some women goes into labour this comes away, sometimes is your telltale sign that labour is coming)

I panicked as I never had this with the girls but I had read and heard about the plug so I instantly screamed for mum.

Mum said "it looks like a plug just call hospital and get checked better safe than sorry"

And that was yet again another time my mum saved me.

I went to the hospital sharply. Midwives on that evening was great I told them my history and said I'm sorry if I'm wasting your time but I don't want history to repeat itself. I did explain that I had no pain but whilst sitting waiting for doctors I felt strange, they put it down to me being anxious which I kind of thought yes possibly.

A couple hours past and a doctor come in and said "Hi Ms Treadwell my team have informed me of your concern, at this stage in your pregnancy there is no way a plug will show."

"Well I'm not convinced and although I don't wish for you to look down there I think you should check."

"No I won't look as don't wish to risk you of an infection "she responded.

"I'm sorry doctor but I'm at my peak time of history and not due to see my consultant for another 9 days please check" I insisted.

This was completely out of character for me to stand my round but something was telling me not to leave that hospital.

I called the emergency number my consultant wrote on my notes as he had requested and no answer, left multiple messages.

After standing my ground and begging a midwife to get the doctor to agree, finally the doctor did.

The doctor was very reluctant to start and to be honest I was pooping it.

Then she gasped took a huge step back and demanded the buzzers to be pushed.
"Please don't tell me what I think you're going to say!?" I said tearing up and shaking.
"I'm so sorry Sian your 2cm dilated, you was right for me to check, we need to get you transferred as soon as possible, we need to tilt you back, please do not stand up." Doctor demanded.
" I knew it!! I screamed "Here we go again!"

Instantly I hated my body more than ever, every inch!
How could this be happening again!!
Was told twice now it wouldn't happen and both times it did at same gestation.
Laying upside down I was again transferred this time was a shorter journey to a more local hospital in Luton. Blue lighted all the way with a midwife in case I delivered on route. Nerve wracking.
Arriving at the hospital on a drip to try slow potentially stop my labour I was whisked into a private delivery suite room.
A lovely midwife was really reassuring that I was in the right place and they will do everything they can to help baby and stop my labour, all I had to do was stay calm.
Sounds easy doesn't … what even was CALM…I lost the meaning of calm.
I tried my best within the circumstance.
I had many medical professions in and out. Lots of medication, drips etc. Within 5 hours of being there I was put on a magnesium drip.

I had never had this before, and have to say the side effects are awful. However the benefits of it does way out the bad effects.
Pros of a magnesium drip is that it helps the baby if born extremely premature to prevent bleeds on the brain.
Which is common so early.
Cons are it makes you feel like your body is on fire. It fades once the drug is stopped but wow it feels like burns, was horrible feeling. Another downside is it lowers blood pressure. I naturally suffer with low blood

pressure in pregnancy.

I had the magnesium and few hours later I felt fine and was looking forward to visitors. Just as my visitors was arriving midwife said I could sit up.

Well minutes before my visitors walked in, I remember saying "I don't feel right"

Next thing I know is vaguely seeing a nurse and my name being called then her arm reaching a buzzer.

I have no recollection of the next part but I remember waking, all my family was there with Mackenzie I hugged her so tight. Then I asked "have I wet myself" one of my fears is passing out and wetting myself, not sure why but it is.

Where I had magnesium it had caused my blood pressure to drop so low I passed out twice.

From here I was fine, had no more effects from it. Relieved.

The main concern was baby boy was ok and given every possible chance to survive.

My family wasn't allowed to stay too long. As the night drew in the midwife shift changed happened.

My new midwife was signed to stay in my room all night occasionally popping out briefly.

Just after midnight I said to her "I feel wet down there"

She looked and said "No it's fine, it's just where your laying down"

Hour later I said "Sorry I'm getting uncomfortable"

Her response "Sian get some sleep"

"I can't its hurting please help me."

Midwife took another look at my pad you are a little damp, I think you have wet yourself"

"i haven't wet myself I don't need a wee, I'm in labour"

"No you're not Sian get some sleep" as she walked out the room.

I pushed the buzzer minutes later "I'm in labour I know I am, I need to PUSH!!" begging for her to listen to me or anyone to listen at this point.

I couldn't fight back the urge of naturally pushing. Next thing I know a doctor came running in, he looked and GUSH!!!

My waters broke literally soaking the medical team at the end of the bed.

I had a sudden feel of relief when waters broke, my contractions had stopped so a nice midwife re stimulated my womb to kick start back up which they did with a vengeance.

I couldn't tell you how many medical staff came rushing in, I remember a neonatal incubator came in with a team preparing for little man.

A doctor demanded a sonographer to come in to check babies position as he was initially breech.

Trying to fight the urges the sonographer confirmed he was breech. I screamed "I'M PUSHING"

Doctor looked. He and his team at the end of the bed looked puzzled. Once my contraction eased I asked what was wrong, Whilst preparing for the next contraction coming….. Doctor responded "looks like his head but it can't it his breech"

Whilst he was standing scratching his head with his team.

I yelled out. Little man came out left to fall on the bed, a little noise so soft and cute as he tried to cry.

The neonatal team lifted him up, the cutest little blondie I ever did see.

Instantly I fell in love all over again.

He was swiftly whisked off whilst I was checked for tears.

Luckily I didn't tear, I was able to shower and refresh myself ready to go see my little man. Felt forever waiting.

I was almost certain that he was going to be ok, especially with all the medication I was given to give him the best chance of survival, which I was never given in previous labours.

Long few hours past, finally I was able to be wheeled to see my little man.

Taking photos of him to send to my family to say he arrived and doing well. He was honestly stunning. Carter 1lb13ozs.

 So tiny my little fighter.

The Neonatal team said I could allow visitors to come see him tomorrow I was so excited for Mackenzie to see her baby brother, my parents to meet him.

 Extremely tired after 8 hours next to little man I needed to go put my head down so I was fresh to spend the day with him meeting his sister.

I was discharged from hospital so the neonatal arranged for me to stay in a local hotel.

As much as I never wanted to leave his side, I knew I needed to rest for the roller coaster I was about to relive.

I manged to get checked in and settled to the hotel around 11:30pm. I Fell asleep around midnight by 2:00am my mobile phone was ringing.

Half asleep "Hello?"

"Hi Ms Treadwell its neonatal team, Carter has taken a turn for the worst we advise you to come in"

In panic "I'm on my way, please don't let him die"

What felt like forever to get to him, I rushed to the side of his incubator "mummy's here baby boy you hold tight" I whispered to him tears streaming.

Carter's alarms kept alarming really loud, red lights flashing, neonatal staff rushing everywhere, it was a whirlwind, I looked up at his monitor and his heart beat had drastically lowered. A nurse held me and I said I had to step outside.

Being guided out into a family room, I looked back, staff rushed to his incubator, I couldn't hold back the tears, repeatedly saying "PLEASE, PLEASE don't let him die!"

In the family room I rang my parents to say Carter had took a turn for the worse, both ends of the phone couldn't speak just cried to each other.

My parents was trying to be strong for me whilst getting ready to come over, unknowing what to tell Mackenzie who was so excited to see her brother.

I was called back in to Carter so I quickly hung up the phone.

Just as I was approaching Carter's incubator his little body crashed and the doctor turned t and I said "I'm so sorry, there's nothing else I can do."

"NO NO NOT AGAIN, PLEASE THERE'S GOT TO BE SOMETHING!" I screamed tears uncontrollable, I fell to my knees.
A midwife ran over to pick me up "PLEASE I BEG YOU, DON'T GIVE UP ON HIM!" begging, praying that he doesn't pass away.
"I NEED HIM"

The neonatal doctor apologized and left the room distraught.

Looking back her job is hardest job, the highs and lows, I'm forever grateful for everything she done to try save my little man.

At the time all I could feel was the pain of losing him.

Little man's body just could not handle the fight, he had multiple drains in his lungs to release the fluid, lots of medication pumped in, his little heart just couldn't cope, he flat lined when his mummy was by his side.

Just like Morgan waited for me.

After a neonatal nurse try to settle me a little as I was hysterical, I went back by Carter's side where he was disconnected from his tubes and wire's and I was allowed to hold him. I wrapped his little body in a cosy blue blanket.

Neonatal nurses gave me a private family room where I could stay until I was ready to allow him to be taken to the morgue, they even had the bag they wanted me to put him in, which I refused and said "I won't be putting him in a bag, you can when I'm gone"

I actually couldn't believe they wanted me to if I'm honest. I managed to get a lock of his hair and hand and foot print which I am forever grateful for.

My parents and Mackenzie arrived, the nurse was great with Mackenzie at explaining what happened and allowed Mackenzie to bath him with her.

Freshly washed and lots if cuddles we left Carter to lay at rest.

Shattered to pieces we headed out the hospital. My dad took Mackenzie off as I just couldn't hold back my emotions. Whilst outside the labour entrance trying to gather myself together I saw multiple women standing heavily pregnant smoking.

I couldn't help but comment to one of them "I done nothing wrong to lose my babies and their you all are smoking killing your babies!" crying letting them know how lucky they are to get to near term but yet they standing smoking harming their little ones with not a care in the world, whilst mine is being taken to a morgue!

Noting more devastating than people not realizing how lucky they are and taking everything for granted.

From the minute you find out your pregnant you are lucky!!

There's women dreaming of being in your position, yet can't be.

I didn't want to go to bed because I didn't want to wake up the next day, I didn't want to talk to anyone let alone see anyone.

I laid in bed hugging little man's neonatal sheet that he laid on in the short time he lived.

Not even 24 hours of Carter's passing I got a message asking what I was doing with Carter's stuff I brought him, and if I would sell it because she (the woman who message) was pregnant.

My blood boiled, still crying, I was struck back at how inconsiderate people can be.

Seriously it's not even been 24 hours and you feel the need to buy my sons stuff, I haven't even buried him and there you are thinking of yourself.

This was a real eye opener.

A few days past I tried to carry on being "normal" as could be especially for Mackenzie as she was far too young to even understand, She knew she had an older sister called Morgan who is the brightest star in the sky, we often before bed used to find the brightest star and blow a kiss. So her way of understanding was Carter has gone to play with Morgan and the angels, now there's two brightest shining stars.

Two kisses a night blown to heaven.

Mackenzie kept me going in the darkest weeks of my life.

She was my reason to keep going, she was my reason to work for the future.

THE FUNERAL

"where do I start?"
"why has this happened again ?"
Head can't focus, mind spinning, no words to speak, crying till no tears left.
 Yet there I was trying to plan a funeral AGAIN.

 I went back to the funeral directors that helped with Morgans funeral,
lovely man he is, he couldn't believe I was back burying another baby.
Both choking up as we was trying to talk figures and plans.

Morgan had a pink little casket, I carried her casket myself into the her
funeral with white gloves on. Head down, holding casket tight, tears
streaming whilst her dedicated song played, there was not a dry eye in sight.
I tried to be so strong that day everyone who came to say goodbye wore
pink in her memory.
 The vicar who christened Morgan at the hospital also did her funeral for
us, Velveteen rabbit verses was read, it's such a beautiful book I will cherish
forever.
 I've never been a confident woman, quite shy, kept myself to myself but at
her funeral I felt I had to do something for her, so I read a poem out, whilst
trying to fight the flowing tears, I stood up and read her a little poem, heart
shattered to a million pieces but it's one thing I am proud I overcome my
shyness, fear and did it for my little girl.
 We then went to where she was being laid to rest, where we threw roses in
as she was lowered.
 I found this very hard to watch and turned around with my head in my
hands crying saying "I can't do this, I don't want to do this"
 You know this has always been an regret of mine, as I feel I turned my
back on her, which I would never ever do, it was the pure emotions of it
being my final goodbye the one goodbye I never thought I would be

saying. The one goodbye I never wanted to say.

 Writing this is bringing back so many raw emotions, even, now I don't have dry eyes, my darling daughter and darling son, I miss you both dearly and not minute in the day goes past where I don't think of you and what life would be like with you. I hope you're playing with the angels and know you're both forever in my heart.
Hardest Good byes.

Do I carry resentment?
Yes
Do I hold hospital accountable?
 yes I feel like both consultants failed me,
 Since my losses I have spoken to many consultants across the world and UK private hospital. All said I should of hade a cervical stitched, placed earlier in my pregnancies, after losing my first.
Then 2nd was labor same time.
 Will touch base back here in a bit.

 Due to the heartbreak when I lost Morgan I didn't have any real say in how her funeral went, as my head just was not capable of the thoughts at all.
All I knew was to request if could a pink casket and I carry her in.
 With Carter it was down to me to plan, hated every moment but this time, I was able to block out certain parts, partly coz I never fully grieved Morgan I blocked.
Is it healthy? Most likely not.
Is it intentionally? Absolutely not! It's just how I got through each day personally,
With having Mackenzie being so small it helped a bit more as I needed to be strong for her, in fact Mackenzie was actually and still is My strength. Distracted with her needs and learning it made the days feel less long.

 The same funeral directors did everything for me they were amazing, blue casket was chosen, Carter was picked up and laid in his casket.
I went to see him and honestly worst thing I ever did. I cannot unsee what I saw. I know some people find comfort in going, but me personally I don't recommend when it's a baby.

 Waiting to be collected for the funeral I stepped outside and wow!! I burst into tears the driveway was filled with the most amazing flowers.
Stunning West ham badge, the most incredible angel wings and many more, was such a beautiful touch.

Carters funeral was very similar to Morgans, I carried him in, stood and read a poem, Mackenzie also read a little poem.
We stood together at the front, there's no one else that day that I needed by my side more, than my little miracle holding my hand, telling me "its ok mummy."
My parents were my strength and held me together most days, they supported every hurdle, every tear. I'm forever grateful for amazing parents.
 After having children and they accidently fall and hurt their knee they cry, it makes you sad, you feel hurt for them. Imagine the pain they felt seeing me broken… Looking back I don't know how they kept strong for me but they did, words just explain how much I appreciate them, love them.

During the service the music was played and there was again not one dry eye in the service.

Morgan and Carter are laid to rest next to each other, very lucky I was able to do this but due to their size it was made possible.
 At the wake we released balloons off with little messages tied to them from anyone that wished to write one. Everyone wore baby blue.
 Nieces and Nephews were incredible with their little memory touches.
Hardest day was made into a touching service.

 The grieving really hits hard after the funeral, I find it's the most loneliest part. That's when reality hits hard.

 When Morgan was laid to rest I did try visit regular, especially on occasions, this was yet to change!
 It wasn't long until people felt the need to trash her grave. From jealously and stirrers at school to now entering adult hood , gossip of my loss flew round and they felt the need to trash a babies grave.
A baby that never effected them , never saw them, had no incompact on their lives.
Yet they felt the need.
My life had been turned upside down yet their hate was brung to her place of rest.
Heartless

After this I found it extremely hard to visit , I don't know why I let them stop me from visiting, as it was all I had left of my baby but they did.
I dread every visit.
A place to sit peacefully was now I anxious dreaded seat.

Do I hate the people for doing it?
No hates a strong word, I petty them for being so heartless, I feel sorry for the fact they listened to hear say from jealous people.
Sorry they felt the need.

After burying Carter with Morgan I tried to visit a lot more but as time passed it became harder and harder. The worry that his would be trashed too if they found out I lost a 2nd baby .
 It made me feel ashamed , I carried so much guilt not being able to visit them. Sometimes it felt they was stolen from me all over again.

At times I feel strong enough to go but then the fear and worry strikes back harder just as I arrive to which sometimes I can only go as far as the layby outside the cemetery, sit cry, blow a kiss and away I drive.

I saw a counsellor in hopes it would help me combat the fear of visiting , instead it built my thought process of the cemetery is where their caskets lay. Their spirits are with me , they are carried in my heart, in my two girls. My home is full of baby angels in their memories, they are spoken about, a little memorial is in our garden.
Special occasions their special candle is lit. Every Christmas they have a special ornament on the tree.

Nothing prepares you for a loss of a child, the days don't get easier.
In time you learn to live with it but you always try to blame or punish yourself.
In time you learn not to be so harsh on yourself and that it was out of your control but theirs one part in your heart and stomach that holds guilt.

7 WHATS INCOMPETENCE CERVIX

 Before we go further.
Please note I am not medically trained this is from my own experiences, advice I was given and my own research.

 Have you ever heard of incompetence cervix before?
No?
Me either until after losing Carter I realized I lost him due to something that was more than "an infection" and could have been prevented, by a cervical suture. Some what of this was proved with the emergency suture that was placed and saved Mackenzie.
Also ask yourself...would you be left with an "infection" for 15+ years without treatment?
I'd be shocked if you your response is yes right now!

From my own research there's three types of sutures.

TRANSABDOMINAL CERVICAL CERCLAGE (TAC)- this is reserved for select people with previous failed transvaginal cerclage. More resulting into caesarean's as this are more permanent.

MACDONALD SUTURE- this can be done in emergency as long as cervix hasn't opened above a certain level and contractions are managed via drip.

SHIRODKAR- Is similar to Macdonald however this one is placed higher up, and preferred to be done between 12-16 weeks.

The above depend on what your consultant recommends. Either from a previous spontaneous loss, or possibly picked up via a scan, usually internal, (sometimes funneling of the cervix can be seen)

Signs of Incompetence cervix:

Pelvic pressure
A new back discomfort
Mild stomach aches although this isn't on all cases, mine wasn't stomach ache.
A change in vaginal discharge
Vaginal bleeding
A history of painless widening of cervix.
There isn't always signs, and sometimes when signs show we convince ourselves it must be normal because no one expects of such premature births.

I always say believe in how you feel, something don't feel right? Go get checked, stand your ground until YOU feel happy.
Been multiple times? Who cares don't allow ANYONE to make you feel a nuisance or that your nuts.
Mothers instinct is always right!

Midwives are incredible but some haven't experienced pregnancy therefore its text book until experience is gained. So just ensure you both are happy with a peace of mind. Most midwives understand your anxiety's and go above and beyond for you, they are incredible!
I had never heard of premature babies let alone incompetence cervix, it's not something that's been spoken about until you experience it an do research yourself then you realize actually a lot of women across the world suffer. We need to raise more awareness and prevent heartaches where we can. Which is why I'm writing this book in hopes I gave save at least one

woman if not thousands.

Since Morgan the medical and awareness of incompetence cervix has strengthened a little, especially with social media.
 I found facebook groups regarding incompetent cervix support for people around the world were savers. They share their experiences, hopes, loses and miracles. It really is incredible.
The support us women can give when experiencing similar is out of this world, we was born to naturally bring life into the world, some of us really have a hard time and these groups are one place full of support and guidance. No judging, no nasty comments.
Just support and love through times of need.

 Although it's sad to read losses and pregnancy fails it is also reality which a lot of us never see, especially on social media, we usually only see happy times for people.
 I always saw people lucky, lucky to fall pregnant fast, lucky to reach to term (even some who smoked and drank throughout, always made me angry that) they never realized how lucky they were.
It made me feel like I was only one who lost, grieving, longing for what they was showing, only one suffering. Even after doing everything right, no drinking/smoking.
Until I found the groups and thought wow incompetent cervix is actually really common, in fact too common and not enough awareness.

Charites like sands, Bliss and Tommys are incredible for support and research. I done a superhero walk in memory of my babies dressed as banana woman a work colleague as bat woman in the pouring of rain after a day of hairdressing, We walk walked from Royston to Cambridge hospital Addenbrookes to deliver handmade crochet hats and blankets from our clients to NICU whilst raising money for Bliss.

A really touching day, I appreciated everyone that helped to make that day possible.

I met my husband and Mackenzie at Addenbrookes welling up with tears of achievement.

When Carter passed I done blow-dry's for a donation which all went to Tommy's charity. This was my stepping stone but into what I love doing.

These charities make a lot of differences to families in NICU, and support to parents.

Looking back to when I had Morgan all the above has come a long way, and I'm hoping this book will raise more awareness.

If I can save at least one person from loosing a baby then I feel like I've achieved. I wouldn't wish what I've been through on anyone.

Your all incredible Women stay strong, know your body, don't pressure yourself, believe in yourself.

8 WELL I NEVER

Took years out to focus on Mackenzie and I, although I never fully wanted to rule out more children, I had started to convince myself that I wouldn't. It was hard to accept but my then life was fully focused on her and myself.

Mackenzie was getting older I never wanted a huge age gap, I carried a lot of pain that not many people understood.

I had started to be able to talk about my losses more which I found a huge strength within to be able to.

As people would say …

"Just the one child?"

"Would you have anymore?"

If I responded "Yes just one" I carried who guilt because that wasn't fair, because my other two passed away why was I not including them…?

then if I responded "No probably not"

I felt like I had to explain myself as they would wait for an explanation.

So to prevent extra emotions to myself I started to just talk about it (without too much details)

In time it became a little easier and sometimes lifted a weight of my shoulders.

When you least expect it things happen.

Do you believe in this saying ?

No? I never did either

But reality is, it's true.

My life started to become ok, and I was loving motherhood. When I met my husband. Of course I was nervous to start again, eventually (months down) I introduced Mackenzie who instantly gravitated which was my biggest fear at time, that fear instantly faded.

A few years passed making lots of memories along the way, a proposal, a wedding then….. the question was popped…..

"More children?"

This was a question I dreaded, I knew It was likely to be asked as he didn't have children, but I just wasn't prepared.

My heart wanting a football team, my head saying not a chance you fail you can't let him go through a loss, you can't carry, you're not able, why put him and his family through it.

Well we sat down and spoke, I voiced all my worries and concerns.

We agreed before jumping into it, because the last thing I wanted was to cause him a loss of a baby, I knew the pain far to well and never wanted to cause him that pain.

We looked into surrogacy but a part of me felt like I had been robbed in my pregnancies and owed it to myself to find out why I couldn't carry to term before I ruled it completely out.

So we decided to go for a private consultation where within minutes the consultant confirmed my research, thoughts and said its sounds like you have incompetence cervix a suture is recommended going forward.

We spoke thoroughly over my history, I also had notes from previous pregnancies that she viewed and her words

"This isn't due to an infection because your tests would of shown one, then would have been treated. Not left 15 years."

I came out feeling content knowing I was right to follow my gut, I knew it was an infection.

My history of exactly 23 weeks pointed in to the direct fact of the cervix. Ask yourself how an infection would know 23 weeks every time forcing that you labor????

I can pretty much think what your answer would be, asking yourself that.

From this we discussed further and without pressure we tried.

I was so nervous of what was to come, but excited I got another try with correct medical guidance.

Would you believe it, it was a busy time in my life, didn't think I was pregnant at all, but I felt odd and thought ill just check…. And there It was a BIG solid positive.

Shocked, felt sick, hyperventilated, mixed emotions of happy, anxious and disbelief.

I instantly that very morning called the GP to request a referral.

Due to covid at the time there was some delays with this but after a bit of push I managed to get seen via a new consultant at the hospital I originally wanted with my son.

My consultant this time was incredible, she was honest but hopeful without giving me false hope.

She knew her knowledge, I actually left having faith, something I never thought I would ever get back.

We knew it was going to be a rocky road ahead but taking every precaution we was willing to proceed.

This was when I found further incompetence cervix facebook groups.

After all the correct checks bloods etc. We set up a plan of action.

I was booked in for my cervical suture at 15 weeks. (I was worried it was being placed a bit too late but that was the next available date)

Then the plan was to hit each milestone and regular two weeks check with my consultant.

Week 15 arrived very quickly, morning sickness I was rife, last time I was this sick I had girls…

Arrived to hospital for my suture to be placed, nervous for the unknown and if it was even possible or going to work, I tried to stay positive, my husband was allowed to stay with me till I was taken down.

Arrived at 7am all checked in, gown on, I awaited surgery.

I was due down in the morning but that day was set back due to lots of emergency's, which I know can't be helped. I was lucky I was able to have this suture so that's what I kept reminding myself to remain positive.

Time went on I was starving, feeling sick from not eating from 8pm the night before, due to needing an spinal block I wasn't allowed to eat.

5:15pm arrived, I heard a nurse come onto the ward calling my name.

Shaking with nerves " I'm here" I responded, grabbing my shoes, wrapping a dressing gown over me ready to be walked to theatre.

Husband whisked off to get some dinner and grab me a MacDonalds for after, good egg he was.

Walking in the theatre was bright white, medical staff everywhere.

I was led to the bed in the middle of the room with huge lights, where a lovely nurse sat with me chatting away trying to keep me calm.

The spinal block was inserted, I was then guided to lay down where the surgery was then performed.

Being awake through it was very odd you don't feel pain, just tugging.

I had a little bleed and was explained there was a little bit of difficulty due to scarring from before, they used a claw grip to pull cervix closed but it tore a little to which consultant controlled the bleeding. but my miracle consultant did it.

I was so relieved, blessed and thankful. I knew I wasn't completely out the woods yet but this was a huge step forward in hope.

I was wheeled into recovery for about half hour then wheeled back to the ward where Hubbie awaited with food.

I was hoping to go home but due to having it done late and slight bleed I had to stay overnight.

Did not sleep a wink, I texted my mum to keep me calm. My mum just gets me, gets my anxiety and knows I'm a wimp when comes to staying in hospital, I was willing to do whatever I needed to keep this baby at the best survival rate.

The following day I was discharged under strict instructions of rest, no lifting, do minimal, No long walks or standing.

A two weekly check till I hit 26 weeks. Then went down to three weeks.

Upon my weekly checks I had internal scan via my consultant herself who checked for funneling and stitch hold, medication was a mistered when need. That being antibiotics if need and cyclogest pessaries.

As left the appointment we always said lets reach week 22 and so on.

Can you believe it I reach 28 weeks then panic set in, all that day I felt tightening's they were becoming regular.

Calling the unit they were great and got me in right away.

The monitor was picking up an irritated uterus, we aren't sure what caused this but it was giving me contractions without actually opening my cervix. The stitch most definitely was doing its job.

As weeks went on I was on edge more and more, although every week was a true blessing, I couldn't help but think it's going to happen again.

Tightening's were still going strong but they wasn't as regular, my cervix was checked, there was no sign it was opening or funneling. Awesome news!!!66

Still on bed rest which I struggle with as I am an active woman,

I just felt lucky, knowing that bed rest was a small price to pay to receive a beautiful baby at the end.

Weeks started being ticked off with celebrations although we had a few alarms of this could be it!

After being checked, it was either resolved, mind put to rest or I had further checkups to ensure we was heading in correct direction.

As I started to hit the 30+ weeks I just couldn't believe it, I was in shock, In fact we all was.

Preparing the baby nursery was just incredible, washing the clothes, setting out the sterilizer's, baby hospital bag these were just huge milestones that I never thought I would ever get to do.

Week 32-34 was very rocky being in and out of hospital due to tightening's, they stopped me in my path even if it was just a walk to the loo.

Laying down my bump would go rock hard.

I attended the maternity unit week 34, again the monitor was picking up contraction a doctor on call that day saw a contraction and agreed with me that we did not want to leave the stitch in rising the chance of tearing.

We all had a chat and came to the conclusion we would remove the stitch and allow mother nature to do what it needed to.

Stitch removal wasn't the easiest but the doctor called for assistance and out it came without any spinal block or pain relief. I was kept down delivery as we all thought I would give birth straight away ....

All of us thinking I would only last a few days!!

You ready for a shock???

I went beyond!!!!
Can you believe it!!

The tightening's eased, they were still there but there wasn't as many. I most certainly was more comfortable, at this stage I was allowed to move about more. Every day I woke saying "think it will be today"

I was completely flabbergasted that I hadn't gone into labor. My main concern was that my labors are quick so I need to ensure I'm near the hospital.

Staying very local. Trying to me more prepared than ever.

35 weeks I started to feel unwell. Earlier in pregnancy I think about week 28 I kept having moments of coming across unwell my heart would race when I ate.

Still to this day I have no idea what caused it, was frequent. When I spoke with medical they put me on a heart monitor and said was normal then other times when they could see racing they said it was my anxiety.

Very odd

Week 35 my blood pressure was raised (not my normal I'm usually the lowest end) heart racing, I went back to hospital.

wavering in and out of hospital as contractions were getting more.
I became very tiring.

 By week 36 I couldn't take anymore I was 3cms, struggling to eat due to racing heart. I never had caffeine or chocolate, I was trying solutions for anxiety like relaxation videos, therapies, keeping mind focused positive.
I was put on a ward to keep eye on my contractions.

 My consultant came to see me and saw I wasn't myself, I was already 3cms dilated so she agreed to help and done a sweep.

 She quoted "my hands have never let me down"
 She stands correct!!!!
That night I went in labor. Early hours contractions became frequent and strong.
 I was examined 7am where I was then taken into delivery as I was 5cms dilated.
I was full of anxiety, nerves but also super excited, I still had fear trying to way out the excitement as Labor itself is scary, the thought of me trying to push a bigger head out freaked me out, I only ever birthed 1-2lbs babies and that made my eyes water. Haha.
I was pooping it.
Midwives were lovely, when arrived in delivery I needed a wee upon going I heavily bled my poor husband trying to mop up as I walked. (sorry to much information, its reality)
I wish my mum was able to come with me and husband, for Mackenzie we knew it needed her grandma and as much normality as possible.
 I came back to the bed and the room started to fill with a few more people. "Sian don't be alarmed, babies heart is dropping we need to deliver her now"
 The most frightening words ever said, "please don't let her die, I can't lose another baby" crying of fear but stopped during the mega contractions, they were brutal coming thick and fast!!
I barely able to deal with the pain.
A doctor insisted I had gas and air. I was very reluctant to have pain relief but I was getting to the point I couldn't bear the pain, wasn't likely to get epidural due to anesthetist's in emergencies.
 "Sian we may need take you to theatre for c-section."
High as a kite I signed all these forms ready, as baby was becoming very distressed.
Doctor said "Sian why we await theatre lets try push baby out naturally, next contraction I need you to push!.

After a few hard pushes the doctor notice a small part of my cervix just wasn't budging causing natural labor to be difficult.

Instantly I was wheeled to theatre where an epidural was put in and doctors said let's try forceps.
By now I was just trying to remain calm.
Few tugs and pulls baby arrived!!
11:55pm

She was placed on me for literally minutes I heard a cry and shouted
 "omg she's alive, she's actually alive!!"
I just couldn't believe it. I had a baby, by this point I wasn't even paying attention to my body, I was just in or for my precious baby and couldn't wait to tell her big sister who was at school.

Wheeled through to recovery my baby girl got to come, I never experienced that before my baby with me the whole time. So in love!

We named her Bexley-banks the cutest little baby weighing 6lbs3ozs
Whilst in recovery I developed a temperature, I was put on antibiotics straight away, baby was also placed on them as was expected sepsis, frightening but all was under control the medical team was on it.
 After a couple of hours we was both wheeled to a ward, Bexley-banks was placed in a little cot with UV lights to help with jaundice. Her levels were high and we had to leave her in this cot as much as possible. In order to reduce the levels.
 Husband by my side which made such a difference Mum and dad waiting by the phone for all the pictures and updates, Mother and father in law full of excited, all just couldn't wait to meet Bexley-banks.
 I felt proud knowing I didn't fail this time, and its all thanks to Dr Hoveyda and her team, Hubbie for helping me push for the care and not leaving my side. Family for being supportive.

After a 3 nights in hospital we was both discharged Monday evening, best feeling in the world, I got to walk (like I pooped myself , due to stitches) out of the hospital with MY BABY!
Even now I can't believe I got to walk out with my baby.
So tiny yet so big compared to my previous, but this time in my arms, this time I had to do the routine, I had full control of mummy world.
 Was it hard? Yes I'd be lying to day a breeze.
Did I love it? Hell yes!!

We didn't tell Mackenzie we was allowed home as we wanted to surprise her, my mum was with me and Bexley – banks till we got discharged as

Hubbie was surprising me at home with full on house decorations to welcome us, tears creeped out my eyes with pure happiness!!
The look on Mackenzie's face with instant love for her sister and 1000's of cuddles was a moment I will ever forget. Super proud sister, to this day her sister title is strong, she's a mini mummy who is absolutely incredible the love between them is pure.
Littlest legs looks up to little legs its just incredible how two miracles come together and make you look at life completely different .

As weeks fly by we all bickered who got to push the pram, done bedtime cuddles and bath. This 2nd miracle so loved by all.

One thing I have to be open about writing this book. Is believe in yourself, believe in your gut.
Yes sometimes your gut can be wrong but very rarely. YOU know your body, medical are incredible there's no denying, but they also don't know how your feeling. YOU know your body, You know how you feel.
Never be frightened to say, actually I'm not insulting your intelligence but I'm feeling x y z and won't settle until rest assured.

I'm glad I researched, paid for private opinions (I felt lucky to of been able to have done this), I emailed consultants across the world, contacted Penny Abatzi @ serum Greece without them I wouldn't have Bexley-banks, without them I'd never of known the reasons for my babies passing and Mackenzie's fight for life.

My advice to you would be….
Believe your gut instinct, doesn't matter if its proved wrong as there will be times it's 100% right and you will wish you listened to it.
Have questions ask them, your not insulting anyone by asking.

I count myself a very lucky woman I have four beautiful children.
 Two children I never thought I would have, every day is a blessing,
Reality is… yes there's hormones, door slamming's, toddler tantrums, sleepiness nights.
Would I change it …NEVER because Miracles happen and they aren't always easy!

To every women ….

YOU are strong
YOU are not a failure

YOU make miracles happen
YOU are the strength between
YOU know your body
YOU are amazing
YOU give life

53

Here's the daily all time question. Not a day passes where I'm not asked this.

"Will you have anymore?"

Honest answer I wouldn't say no but of course complications follow…

Therefore …..

9 TO BE COTINUED....

ABOUT THE AUTHOR

Born in 1988 grew up in Hertfordshire, studied at Sheredes school in Hoddesdon. School years weren't the easiest.

Fully focus was on anything to do with hair and beauty, that's where the true passion lied, dreams were focused.

Having a baby early did slow career down but determination was carried through which made achievements more appreciated.

Family being the main support to ensure dreams possible

Sian has always been loyal, honest and focused on what she wants from life, after hitting plenty of hurdles and pauses she has overcome leading her strength to strength.

A saying she believes got her through many tough times …

> Through the storm to the rainbow.
> No storm lasts forever.

Whilst her full focus is her girls, her other focus is raising awareness, further support for incompetence cervix, baby loss and finding mummy again whilst grieving.

You are not alone, reach out.

Wishing you all the best & baby fairy dust

xxxx